Ayurveda: A History of Healing

HIMAJA MADDALI

Contents

Introduction

Ayurveda: A History of Healing delves into the ancient medical system that originated in India, exploring the fundamental basics before evaluating key concepts that are pivotal in this alternative system of healing. It examines the three foundational texts, the herbs used, the struggles and conflicts between Ayurveda and Western medicine, and more. My journey into the rich history of Ayurveda was fueled by my curiosity of its practices and treatment, which differed greatly to the western system of medicine that is predominant across the world. I decided on writing a book about Ayurveda as often, it is not spoken about or taught in school, even in India. I wanted to enhance my knowledge and shed light upon a system that has existed for years, providing insights regarding the holistic approach of healing which emphasizes the importance and the interconnectedness of body, mind, and spirit. Ayurveda provides a comprehensive diagnosis that is beyond symptom treatment, propelling for a balanced approach to wellness, based on long term maintenance of health through healthy dietary and lifestyle practices. Additionally, this book also includes first hand information from a professional in the field of Ayurveda, an Ayurvedic doctor, who learned about this system extensively for years, imparting her knowledge to me, during an interview I conducted. If you are someone who seeks to deepen your understanding in Ayurveda, like me, this book provides the necessary details, consolidating information from various sources, and this book may even encourage you to

embrace Ayurvedic practices and incorporate it in your own life.

Chapter 1: The Origin of Ayurveda

Ayurveda is a system of medicine that originated thousands of years ago in India, and it is derived from the Sanskrit terms 'Ayur' and 'Veda', which translates, verbatim, to the knowledge of life. This system of healing is based heavily on the concept of balance in all aspects of life, such as diet, lifestyle, and thoughts to maintain good health. Knowledge of Ayurveda hence allows one to learn how to have balance in one's body, mind and soul, depending on each individual, as well as to bring about appropriate changes in one's life to maintain this balance.

To learn further about this system of healing that dominated much of India, it is important to understand the origin of Ayurveda. Initially, this knowledge was passed orally and documented in Sanskrit over five thousand years ago. The origin of this system of medicine can be traced back to the Vedas, ancient sacred scriptures of the Hindu religion. More specifically, the Atharvaveda, or the fourth Veda, contains concepts and mantras that are specifically referenced and mentioned by Charaka and Sushruta, physicians and ancient doctors who were instrumental in pioneering the system of Ayurveda.

Although Lord Brahma, the creator of the universe, is said to be the disseminator of this practice, according to Hindu Mythology, Lord Dhanvantari, the physician of devas, is said to be the god of Ayurveda, as referenced in the Puranas. Lord Dhanvantari is said to be an avatar of Lord Vishnu. Lord Vishnu, as an incarnation of Dhanvantari, was born out of the milky, churning ocean, holding a container filled with the amrita elixir (which grants immortality) that gods and demons sought out, and ayurveda in the other. He was born to King Dhanwa as the King of Kasi, where he learned the science of Ayurveda from sage Bharadhwaja, more particularly, the surgical aspect. Dhanvantari, as Divodasa passed on this knowledge to his disciples, which included Sushruta. Thus, at the start of many Ayurvedic works, veneration and prayers are recited towards Lord Dhanvantari.

Ancient sages, Charaka, Sushruta and Vagbhata then compiled their knowledge and the learnings of the system of Ayurveda into comprehensive works. Charaka authored the "Charaka Samhita", Sushruta for the "Sushruta Samhita", and Vagbhata was known for the "Ashtanga Hridaya", which are indispensable and foundational texts in the field of Ayurveda. Ayurveda is fundamentally based on these three texts and is known as the "Brihatrayi" or "The Great Triad". Minor classics, referred to as the "laghu trayi" or the "Lesser Triad/Trio" comprised of "Madhava Nidana" written by Acharya Madhavakara, "Sharangadhara Samhita" by Acharya Sharangadhara, and "Bhavaprakasha" written by Acharya Bhavamishra.

Chapter 2: Principles of Ayurveda

The Doshas

According to Ayurveda, the five elements, or the Mahabhutas, constitute the world. This includes Akash, which is ether or space; Jala, which is water; Prithvi, which is earth; Teja, which is fire; and Vayu, which is air. An amalgamation of all these elements forms the Tridoshas, which are energies that control a person's physical, mental and emotional well-being, contributing to maintaining balance and harmony in our bodies. The three doshas are named Vata, Pitta and Kapha, and every person is said to have a unique and distinct proportion of each dosha, playing a pivotal role in the cognizance of one's mental and physical constitution as well as health and well being.

Vata

'Vata' is defined as 'to blow like the wind'. This dosha is predominantly made up of the two elements, air and ether, and the qualities associated with Vata are light, mobile, dry, cold and rough. Vata governs all movements and mobility in the body, including the circulation of blood, excretion, egestion and the removal of waste substances, the movement of thoughts in the brain, blinking, inhalation, and exhalation. Those who are proportionately more Vata are said to be energetic and enthusiastic, flexible, sensitive and creative. Typically, they appear to be slim and delicately built, with dry skin and fine hair. They speak quickly and have high fluctuating and temperamental moods.

Vata subcategories

The Vata dosha is further segregated into its five subdoshas: Prana, Samana, Vyana, Udana and Apana. Prana Vata, or forward-moving air, regulates processes such as inhalation and deglutition (swallowing), sneezing, and belching. It determines motivation and bridges one with one's soul and inner self. Samana Vata, or equalizing air, handles digestion and assimilation. Furthermore, it aids in the balance of Prana and Apana, maintaining stability and balance within our body. Vyana Vata, or outward moving air, governs the veins, joints, muscles and nerves originating from the heart, allowing the flow of different liquids, such as perspiration, contraction and extension, and more. Udana Vata, or upward moving air, is the energy that resides in the face and throat, in charge of facial expressions, speech, and exhalation. Udana is responsible for transporting the mind from a state of being awake to sleep. It also plays a role in life after death. It rises from our body and directs us to the various universes based on our willpower, energy, and the karma that flows through it. It is, therefore, responsible for separating our existence and rising above the external world (Yoga is primarily associated with the development of Udana). Lastly, Apana Vata, or the downward moving air, controls processes such as urination, menstruation, waste removal, and more. Apana grounds the consciousness, in contrast to other subcategories of Vata, such as Udana. When aggravated, it results in decay and breakdown, and thus, Vata imbalances are typically solved by addressing and making Apana the focus.

Pitta

'Pitta' means digestion or 'that which digests', and it is made up of the elements of fire and water, with qualities such as heat, light, oily, sour, sharp and spreading. It accounts for all the metabolic activity in the body that releases heat. It deals with energy and heat transformation. While it is commonly linked with just digestion, it is also responsible for other organ systems. The body of the Pitta type is of medium build and muscular, with a golden-tanned skin complexion and a tendency to have freckles. They often perspire heavily and are said to have prematurely graying hair. Their personality is described to be confident. They possess high self-assurance and qualities such as passion, competitiveness, warmth, and fierceness, as well as outstanding leadership due to their tendency to take charge.

Pitta subcategories

Sadhaka

Sadhaka controls the brain and the heart, dealing with the 'digestion' of emotions, experiences and stress. It is essential in keeping the mind alert and observant and is responsible for removing melancholy from the heart. An imbalance in Sadhaka can prevent happiness and can cause a build-up of emotions as people struggle to find a way to release them.

Bhrajaka

Bhrajaka is in charge of the skin and the area of touch, giving protection, aiding circulation, controlling temperature, and dealing with external changes. Therefore, an imbalance of Bhrajaka causes various skin problems such as dryness, acne, etc.

Panchaka

Panchaka rules the stomach, although it is also present throughout the digestive tract, where this process takes place. Out of all the subdoshas, Panchaka is the most important due to the importance of digestion in Ayurveda. It governs the digestive fire, known as 'jatar agni' or 'panchaka agni', which plays a major role in the breakdown of the food consumed. Imbalance in this subdosha can lead to digestive issues such as lazy bowel syndrome, slow digestion, hyperacidity, bloating, and appetite issues.

Alochaka

Alochaka governs the sense of sight. It also gives rise to the perception of what is correct and what is incorrect. An imbalance can lead to problems in vision and eye infections.

Ranjaka

Ranjaka is present in the internal organs, navigating the formation of plasma and blood, and responsible for the flow throughout the body. Ranjak means coloring agent (understood to be hemoglobin of blood) in Sanskrit and it is in charge of the change of plasma into blood. It also controls the coloration of stool, urine, eyes, hair and skin color. If out of balance, problems in the skin and early graying of hair are brought about.

Kapha

The third dosha Kapha comprises earth and water with characteristics such as heavy, steady, slow, cold, soft, thick and solid. Kapha gives strength, form and shape and furthermore provides hydration to cells, moistens the joints and skin. The body of the Kapha type is solid, wide and strong, with thick bones. Additionally they have long, thick hair with fair skin. They are calm and serene, with slow reaction times. Kapha is also associated with love, and Kapha types tend to be caring and compassionate.

Kapha subcategories

The five subdoshas of Kapha are Avalambak, Tarpaka, Shleshaka, Bodhaka and Kledaka. Avalambak Kapha, which translates to "hold", resides in the upper thorax, holding the organs, particularly, the respiratory system, including the lungs, and its substructures. Tarpaka Kapha, present in the head, sustains the nervous systems, associated with the cerebrospinal fluid, which is present in the gaps of the brain and the spinal cord. Shleshaka Kapha is the lubrication of the human joints, present throughout the entire body, which allows mobility in the joints. Bodhaka Kapha, situated in the mouth, throat and tongue helps in recognising tastes. Kledaka Kapha is found in the stomach region, governs the discharge and production of substances that mixes with the food we consume to aid with the process of digestion. Additionally, it is a form of defense by not allowing the acidic substances in the stomach from damaging the gut.

Prakriti

In a person's constitution, a person can be Vata, Pitta or Kapha dominated, meaning that one dosha is more prevalent, as compared to the other two, Prakriti is unique to each person and is said to remain unchanged throughout one's life. As explored, each dosha gives rise to characteristics and physical and mental attributes. Charaka and Sushrate have categorized people into seven types depending on the prevalence of the doshas. The seven Prakriti are those with a dominant Vata dosha (Vata prakriti), Pitta, Kapha, Vata-Pitta, Vata-Kapha, Pitta-Kapha, and Vata-Pitta-Kapha (balanced doshas).

Srotas- the body channels

The Tridoshas move throughout the body through channels known as Srotamsi. These channels flow throughout our body, in the respiratory, cardiovascular, reproductive, nervous system, and more. The Maha Srotas, or the gastrointestinal tract is the biggest Srotas, and the smallest is found in individual cells. They are porous in nature, allowing the exchange of nutrients and oxygen into the body with carbon dioxide out of the body. Srotamsi allow for the transportation of blood, absorption of nutrients needed by the body, and the removal of waste substances from the body, and essential body functions to occur. Blockages in these channels can lead to dire consequences and diseases.

Imbalances of Doshas

Each dosha governs different parts and processes of the body and has certain qualities associated with it. Vata controls movement, Pitta is in charge of metabolic activity, and Kapha maintains the balance of fluids and the structure of the body. Naturally, imbalances in each dosha result in problems experienced by the body as directed by the qualities of each dosha.

Vata imbalances can manifest in the form of dry and rough hair, nails and skin; dark blotches on the skin; and cracked lips. It can cause issues in mobility, such as paralysis, and impact body processes, such as respiration, digestion, and circulation (this can result in cold extremities, such as the hands and feet). Cardiac problems, breathlessness, cough, hiccups, constipation, diarrhea and bloating are also a few other symptoms experienced. Imbalances in Vata can also impact our mental health, causing anxiety, fear, struggle to focus, difficulty in sleeping and mood swings.

Pitta imbalances cause redness in the eyes and severe digestive issues like acid reflux, gastritis, heartburn, extreme hunger and thirst as well as skin diseases including rashes, acne, rednesses and inflammation. Mental impacts are also seen, with an increased tendency for frustration, anger, aggressiveness and competitiveness.

Kapha imbalances can cause cold, congestion, allergies, heaviness in the stomach, slow digestion, weight gain, nausea, excessive production of saliva and mucus. Additionally, people could experience heightened feelings of drowsiness, lethargy, and sluggishness. Thus, a plethora of imbalance symptoms are seen, and Ayurvedic diagnosis identifies which Dosha is the cause of an ailment or disease.

Balance, Diet and Lifestyle

The concept of balance is central in Ayurveda, and Ahara (diet) and Vihara (lifestyle) are key to achieving balance in one's life. There are two concepts: Pathya, which is beneficial to one's Prakriti or constitution, thus promoting health, and Apathya, which is harmful and ill suited to a person, resulting in imbalances. There are certain dietary guidelines to be followed to maintain good health. Some include eating on time, eating when hungry, and, according to one's Prakriti, practicing good hygiene and eating food which belongs to six taste groups (described below). In addition to this, the quantity of food consumed is also important. According to Sushrata and Vagbhata, if the capacity of the stomach is split into four different sections, ideally, two parts should be solid food, one should be liquid, and one should be empty to allow for Vata movement. A particular order in which food is consumed is also beneficial to Ahara. Begin with Guru (heavy), Madhura (sweet) and (Snigdha) oily foods, followed by Amla (sour) and Lavana (salty). Finally, end with Ruksha (dry), Katu (pungent or spicy) and Tikta (bitter) foods. This sequence ensures that the jatar Agni, the digestive fire, enhances the body's capability to effectively use the nutrients present in the food we consume. Additionally, it is important to understand the foods that are incompatible to one's body; known as Viruddhahara, which is a diet regime that prevents metabolism because of the wrong combination of foods, incorrect timing of consumption and at wrong proportions. It can lead to consequences such as indigestion, impotency, fainting, anemia, skin diseases, etc.

A regular routine fosters a sense of stability and balance. Lifestyle is essential in treating long-term diseases and is established through a balanced routine that aligns with one's Prakriti. A daily routine, known as dinacharya, encourages the development of a way of life that is in tune with the environment or nature. Certain practices such as waking up early in the morning between 4:00 AM and 5:30 AM, drinking water to clear out the toxic substances, practicing yoga, and regular exercise are key to establishing a healthy dinacharya and a balanced life. Ritucharya, on the other hand, is a seasonal regimen that adjusts and adapts one's routine and habits according to the various months of the year in order to continue to maintain balance. In spring, it is advised to have bitter and hot foods, and avoid salty, sour and sweet meals. In summer, cold, sweet, oily and liquid foods should be consumed while spicy, hot, salty foods should be kept away as Pitta levels would be exacerbated. During the winter, Vata would be heightened, and thus, hot, sweet, sour foods should be consumed; meanwhile, in autumn, bitter diets are preferred.

Ayurveda does not restrict optimal health to just one's physical well-being. It is primarily centered around attaining harmony and balance within the individual and between a person and nature, the environment they exist in. Ayurveda encourages a way of living that considers balance, emotional and physical health, and harmony in all aspects of life to achieve ideal health.

Chapter 3: Charaka Samhita and Ashtanga Hridaya

The Charaka Samhita and Ashtanga Hridaya are the foundational texts of Ayurveda. They are considered the oldest and most credible sources of information, providing comprehensive and in-depth knowledge regarding the principles and practices of Ayurvedic medicine.

Charaka Samhita

The existing version of the Charaka Samhita is believed to be authored by the great Maharshi Charaka in the first century CE. Aside from being a wealth of medical knowledge, it also provides insights into social and daily life in ancient India. Medical geography, or the human and environment interactions resulting in diseases and health conditions, is said to originate from the Greek physician Hippocrates; the Charaka Samhita was written eons before and speaks extensively on medical geography.

According to research, the Charaka Samhita was written centuries before by Agnivesha, a disciple of sage Atreya Punarvasu, the descendant of the

Saptarishi Atri Agnivesha, who taught Ayurveda to his disciples after learning the knowledge imparted by sage Bharadhwaja. Each of sage Atreya's disciples Agnivesha, Bhela, Jatukarna, Parashara, Harita, and Ksharapani, created a samhita (a compilation). However, the one written by Agnivesha, the Agnivesha Samhita, is the most respected, profound, comprehensive, and unparalleled in depth and scope. Charaka then explicated and fine-tuned the Agnivesha Samhita, forming the Charaka Samhita.

The Charaka Samhita is made up of 120 chapters, divided into eight subsections, the ashtanga sthanas, namely, Sutra, Nidana, Vimana, Sarira, Indriya, Chikitsa, Kalpa, and Siddha. Each sthana consisted of several chapters and addressed several different aspects. However, Charaka mainly focused on diagnosing diseases and considered Ayurveda to be a holistic healthcare system. He specifically handled topics such as human anatomy, taxonomy of diseases, the workings and problems experienced by the body (according to the doshas), and more.

Sutra Sthana contains the principles and the fundamental concepts of Ayurveda, providing the foundational structure to understand health, disease, and treatment procedures in thirty chapters, separated into seven quadrates or sapta chatushkas. Nidana Sthana comprises eight chapters with information pertaining to diseases, focusing on the diagnosis, including the causation, symptoms, and pathogenesis. It provides guidelines for identifying several ailments based on clinical observations and diagnostic techniques. Vimana Sthana delves into the different factors that influence disease and health, addressing bodily factors, tastes, qualities of substances, body channels, and specific diseases. It gives insights into the causes, symptoms, and treatments of different health conditions. Sarira Sthana delineates the physiology and anatomy of the human body according to Ayurvedic principles. It describes the functions and structures as well as the interconnectedness of bodily systems, important organs, and tissues. Indriya Sthana deals with observing symptoms and their significance in maintaining health, predicting one's lifespan and dealing with reduced life expectancy. It delves into the functions of the different senses, their role in perceiving the external environment, and covers a significant topic regarding the damage to the sensory system. Chikitsa Sthana focuses on therapeutic principles, the maintenance of health and the prevention and management of different illnesses and diseases. The word 'Chikitsa' itself translates to treatment or therapy. It includes detailed descriptions of medicinal herbs and the process of preparation of medicinal rasayana medications. Rasayana is nutrition at all stages. It nourishes and rejuvenates the body and strengthens the immune system, preventing disease from occurring. Kalpa Sthana explores the formulations and procedures for therapeutic interventions such as Vamana (emesis or vomiting), Virechana (purgation or laxative), as well as other detoxification treatments. It elucidates the preparation, administration, and effects of medicinal substances used in these therapies. Siddha Sthana is concerned with concepts connected to rejuvenation, longevity, and the prevention of diseases. It includes information regarding Rasayana therapies, methods to maintain health and well-being, and methods for strengthening energy levels, longevity and endurance.

Charaka Samhita emphasizes promotive and preventive measures. It delves into the usage of dravyas, or substances such as herbs, minerals, and natural substances used for medicinal purposes and therapeutic treatment, aiming to promote holistic health by balancing individual Prakriti. It also discusses the ethics and basics of medical practice.

Ashtanga Sangraha and Hridaya

Acharya Vaghbata was the author of one of the great treatises of Ayurveda, Ashtanga Hridaya. He also authored the Ashtanga Sangraha, which is considered the more challenging of the two texts in terms of ability to possess a comprehensive understanding. These books appear to have been influenced by the Charaka Samhita and the Sushrata Samhita. Ayurvedic books tend to be highly detailed and convoluted, making them difficult to comprehend; however, the Ashtanga Hridaya contains the "essence," creating a balance between brevity and complexity.

The author states that, "By churning the great ocean of medical science, a great store of nectar by the name Astanga Sangraha was obtained. From that store of nectar has arisen Astanga Hridaya[m] for the benefit of less intelligent people". This denotes the fact that Vagbhata has analyzed and drawn excerpts, quoting and referencing from different works prior to the existence of the Astanga Sangraha and Hridaya, creating a much more straightforward, comprehensible and lucid text. This type of text is known as the Prakarana Grantha.

The name can be divided into two parts: 'Ashta,' which translates to eight, 'anga,' which means branches, and 'Sangraha,' or compilation. This, therefore, means a 'compilation of the eight branches of Ayurveda.' The eight branches of Ayurveda are known as Kaya, Bala, Graha, Urdhwanga, Shalya, Damshtra, Jara, and Vrisha.

Kaya Chikitsa deals with general medicine and treatment of different diseases affecting the body organs and systems. Bala Chikitsa specializes in the care and treatment of children, including their physical and mental health; this branch closely resembles modern paediatrics. Graha Chikitsa deals with the treatment and diagnosis of psychiatric disorders and mental illnesses. Urdhvanga Chikitsa focuses on diseases related to the ears, nose, throat, and eyes, or more specifically, ENT and ophthalmology. Shalya Chikitsa includes surgical techniques and procedures for tending to various illnesses that need physical intervention. Damstra Chikitsa is the study of toxins, their effects on the body, and their procedures for treatment. Jara Chikitsa, or geriatrics is concerned with the health and problems of elderly individuals, and methods to promote a longer lifespan. Vrishya Chikitsa deals with sexual health, fertility treatments, and rejuvenation therapies.

Comparison between the Ashtanga Sangraha and Ashtanga Hridaya

The Ashtanga Sangraha is made up of 6 sthanas with 150 chapters, whereas, while the Ashtanga Hridaya also comprises 6 sthanas, it is only 120 chapters in total. The 6 sthanas are Sutra, covering the basic principles, preventive measures and more; Shareera, which includes anatomy and physiology; Nidana, contains etiology, pathology, symptoms and prognosis; Chikitsa, has medicines and diet; Kalpa, comprises of elimination therapies or panchakarma and formulations; and Uttara, which has the various branches of Ayurveda. While both texts cover similar topics, variation is seen in the number of chapters and depth of coverage. The Ashtanga Hridaya is therefore noted for being a more concise and simplified version compared to Ashtanga Sangraha.

The Charaka Samhita and Ashtanga Hridaya are essential scriptures of Ayurveda, offering a rich and detailed exploration of Ayurvedic medical principles and practices. While Charaka Samhita primarily specializes in the Kaya Chikitsa, and Sushrata Samhita in Shalya, the Ashtanga Sangraha or Hridaya covers all the eight branches of Ayurveda, exploring each in an understandable manner.

Chapter 4: Ayurveda and Surgery: The Sushruta

The Sushruta Samhita, written by the physician and surgeon, and the father of Indian surgery, sage Sushruta, belongs to the foundational texts of Ayurveda. It provides an advanced and in-depth understanding of surgery in ancient India. This book is believed to have been written around the 6th century BCE, serving to be one of the oldest surgical treatises in the world, providing pivotal information on the understanding of anatomy. The book is written in a very structured way, detailing descriptions of surgical procedures, presenting surgical procedures and postoperative care, displaying an approach to medicine that has influenced ancient and modern surgical practices. Sushruta also considered the hand to be the most important instrument, a concept that is pertinent in modern surgical practice.The hand is an important instrument for the surgeon. Sage Sushruta also detailed dissection preparation using a corpse, detailing how studies should be conducted.

This book is composed of 184 chapters, divided into two parts: the Purvatantra and the Uttaratantra, where the first part is further divided into five books, namely, sutrasthana, nidanasthana, sarirasthana, kalpasthana, and cikitsasthana, with 120 chapters in total. The first section deals with the basic principles, surgical instruments, diet, surgical measures, medications and drugs. The second subsection consists of the cause of the disease, the development and symptoms of surgical diseases. The third part comprises chapters filled with information regarding anatomy, physiology, and embryology. The fourth component covers the management of surgical diseases, and principles of handling medical conditions such as emergencies during childbirth. Additionally, Sushruta provided recommendations on pain management during surgery. He advised using wine as an anesthetic to reduce the feeling of awareness and pain before performing operations. This is one of the earliest known references to the use of anesthesia in medical history, highlighting Sushruta's advanced understanding of patient care during surgery. Additionally, the part includes Panchakarma therapies, which are a set of five detoxification and purification treatments used in Ayurveda to purify the body of toxins and achieve balance and harmony within the body. The final subsection elaborates on toxicology, dealing with the concept of poison in different contexts, such as animal poison, and food poisoning, detailing the management of poison as well. The second section, the Uttaratantra, details surgical techniques and procedures, with detailed descriptions of surgical instruments, which formed the basis of modern instrument development. Sushruta's text includes detailed instructions on the types of incisions, suturing techniques, and the importance of precise surgical methods. The well thought out structure of the book covers a range of medical procedures, displaying the advanced nature of this approach to medicine. This structure comprehensively provides information in a detailed manner.

How has Sushruta contributed to surgical practice?

The surgical knowledge contained in the Sushruta Samhita significantly influenced medical practices in ancient India and beyond. This text has been translated into Arabic and Latin, spreading to other civilizations and countries, proving the advanced surgical knowledge contained within this text. Sushruta also emphasized the influence of holistic healthcare, detailing postoperative care, the use of anesthesia during surgery, healthy diet and balance. His detailed descriptions of surgical procedures, such as rhinoplasty and various methods of wound treatment, laid the foundation for modern plastic and reconstructive surgery. The method described by Sushruta is used and is referred to as the "Indian flap" method.

The Sushruta Samhita's contributions to surgery display the advanced medical knowledge of ancient India. Its influence on both ancient and modern surgery highlights the relevance of Ayurveda in the history of medicine. His detailed descriptions of surgical instruments, procedures, and the emphasis on both textual and practical knowledge shows a holistic approach to healthcare that remains relevant, even today.

Chapter 5: Ayurvedic Diagnostics and Treatments

Ayurvedic approaches diagnostics and treatments of health and disease comprehensively, highlighting the importance in the balance of mind, body, and spirit, using observation and examinations for diagnosis. According to Ayurveda, the primary reason for illnesses and maladies experienced in the body is due to an imbalance between the three fundamental doshas: Vata, Pitta, and Kapha.

Nidana Panchaka translates to "fivefold causative factors" It is a term used in Ayurveda to denote the five components that are required in comprehending the causative factors and diagnosis of an ailment.

Nidana are the factors that are responsible for the disease. Understanding Nidana allows personalized treatment plans tailored to individual Prakriti, allowing preventive care through early recognition.

Purvarupa is the prodromal symptoms, the first symptoms experienced by an individual. These are the signs exhibited by people prior to being afflicted, indicating the manifestation of ailments. Samanya Purvarupa are the unspecified prodromal symptoms, which provides an indicator for upcoming diseases but do not reveal the doshas that cause the disease. Vishesha Purvarupa are specific premonitory symptoms as it reveals the doshas responsible for disease manifestation in one's body. Shareera are the preliminary symptoms that only affect at a physical level. In contrast, Manasa are those that afflict at a mental level, and Shareera-Manasa are those symptoms that impact individuals both physically and mentally. Purvarupa is important as it contributes to early diagnosis, which helps in efforts to cure the illness before it progresses into a more dangerous situation.

Rupa are the manifested symptoms. These symptoms appear and evolve during the ailment and are extremely important for the diagnosis. The Rupa of the illnesses is seen when the doshas are aggravated and the disease forms.

Samprapti is pathogenesis, or how a disease develops within the body. The stages of disease are outlined in six steps.

- Sanchaya stage- the buildup of toxins and doshas accumulate in their respective areas, causing an imbalance of doshas in an individual's body.

- Prakopa stage- the Doshas become aggravated and they are not contained at their sites, and begin to overflow.

- Prasara stage- the dissemination and spread from the original sites through the body's channels, the Srotas.

- Sthana-samshraya stage- the doshas localize and settle in a specific organ.

- Vyakti stage- the disease has fully manifested, with noticeable and visible symptoms.

- The last expression of the disease, the Bheda stage- the progression of the disease into the chronic stage, resulting in complications and irreversible damage in the tissues structure and function.

Upashaya and Anupashaya help in the treatment of diseases which have hidden symptoms. Upashaya identifies relieving factors that provide crucial information regarding the nature of disease, allowing diagnosis through observation and trial and error methods. Anupashaya are the non-relieving factors, which cause aggravation, exacerbating the imbalance in the body and worsening the disease. Understanding and identifying Anupashaya is important in order to reduce and remove these factors in order to heal and restore balance. Upashaya treatments include introducing changes in dietary habits, particular herbal therapies, lifestyle modifications, and therapies to relieve symptoms and re-establish the balance in the body, aiding in the healing process.

Other common diagnosis methods involve examinations of the pulse rhythm and strength, tongue color and texture, iris, face reading for identifying dosha imbalances, Ahara and Vihara (diet and lifestyle), and questioning the patients regarding their family and medical history, health, symptoms and more.

Ayurvedic methods focus on diagnosing and treating health and disease holistically, emphasizing the concept of balance. Through the Nidana Panchaka treatment, diseases are effectively diagnosed in this system of medicine.

Chapter 6: Key Herbs in Ayurveda

Herbs have been an integral part of one's lifestyle since the Vedic period. In Ayurveda, plants play a pivotal role, forming the backbone of Ayurvedic medicine, offering a natural and holistic approach to health and healing. They are mentioned extensively in the seminal texts of Ayurveda, such as the Charaka Samhita, with comprehensive explanations of the medicinal purposes.

According to the Charaka Samhita, drugs don't function solely due to their inherent qualities (gunas). Rather, their effectiveness is also dictated by their physical nature as well as how they interact with the body's systems (Dhatu). The specific effects of a drug depends on multiple factors, such as the potency, the target site, or where the drug acts, the timing, and the method of application.

In Ayurveda, Dravyaguna Vijnana deals with food and medicine and its scope includes the application of plant drugs. The term "ousadhi" refers to medicinal plants, taken from the Sanskrit word "osadha," which implies a transformative process with a beneficial outcome. More specifically, "osadha" can connote to "one that removes pain" or "one that brings about a beneficial change." This suggests that plants possess an energy that helps in life processes and helps in restoring balance, therefore making them effective and efficient for treating diseases and illnesses. Ousadhi comprises all stages, from the plant source to the processed drug. Different parts of plants, such as roots, bark, heartwood, and fruits, are used, depending on their particular properties and processed into medicinal drugs. In traditional texts, additional plant materials like internal and external skins, and scrapings, are also noted for their medicinal uses. It is used till date and many people in parts of the world believe they see the benefits written in the book, some proven in research.

Ashwagandha in Ayurveda is used as a Rasayana, an herbal tonic that nurtures a more youthful mental and physical state and increases happiness. While it is used for various treatments, it is specifically and commonly used as a tonic to calm the nerves, as a sedative. As an ayurvedic herb, it holds a predominant position, serving to be one of the most important and revered herbs. It is available mostly as a churna, or a fine powder that can be mixed with ingredients such as honey, milk and water. It improves brain and memory power, and nerve function as well as enhances reproductive balance. As an adaptogen, it aids in the body's strength for stress. It is used for malnutritioned children, frailty due to age, insomnia, nervous breakdown, inflamed joints (applied as a paste) and more.

Turmeric is another highly valued herb. It has several medicinal properties, according to Ayurveda, such as increasing strength and energy of the body, enhancing digestion and aiding in arthritis pain. It contains anti-inflammatory, antioxidant, and antimicrobial properties and is frequently utilized to reduce inflammation, and enhance the body's natural healing processes. Additionally, it is used as a treatment method for respiratory conditions such as asthma and other chronic diseases including liver disorders, rheumatism, and diabetic wounds. Its active compound, curcumin, has been studied for its health benefits,including in its role in preventing and managing chronic diseases such as heart diseases and diabetes. Since forever, my mother has always added turmeric in multiple dishes while cooking, such as dal, curries, and chutneys.

Amla, or the Indian gooseberry has also gained a prominent place in Ayurveda and it has several benefits. It is known for its ability to improve immunity, due to its antibacterial properties which aids in improving the body's immune system, as well as increasing the body's white blood cell count. Additionally, it is important in hair care. Amla is also a popular ingredient in several shampoos produced in India– and is often found in shampoos in Indian households.. Due to its high level of antioxidant and iron content, it helps reduce hair fall, which is why it is used in shampoos. Amla is also known to reduce stress, support respiratory health, and its role in digestion. It is beneficial for the eyes as it contains carotene, which is helpful for vision-related conditions. Furthermore, Amla is celebrated for its positive effects on skin care.

Another herb, Tulsi, is regarded as extremely important in Indian culture and possesses many health benefits. In Ayurveda, it's used to treat several complications such as skin conditions such as acne, by killing bacteria; digestive issues; and respiratory problems such as tuberculosis and bronchitis. According to research, tulsi has the ability to boost the function of the immune system, protect cells, and battle cancer, attributed to its high content in eugenol. Furthermore, it lowers cholesterol, slows skin aging, and helps heart health as it contains antioxidants such as eugenol and vitamin C. Tulsi can help in kidney stones treatment as it can act as a mild diuretic and dissolve the stones. It also helps in decreasing fever, and reducing pain caused by headaches and migraines.

Ayurvedic formulations often combine several herbs and minerals to enhance their therapeutic effects, customized to the individual's Prakriti and the herbs are revered for their role in preventive health care. Ayurveda underscores the importance of maintaining balance in order to prevent illnesses and diseases. The herbs provide a natural and holistic approach to health and healing. Due to their diverse properties and actions, Ayurvedic herbs aid the body's ability to heal and maintain balance.

Ayurvedic herbs are often incorporated into one's lifestyle and diet, frequently without your knowledge.Various herbs are used daily, and several people are unaware of the fact that these herbs are even Ayurvedic. Despite not knowing extensively about this ancient system of medicine, Ayurveda plays a pivotal role in everyday life.

Chapter 7: Can Ayurveda and Western Medicine Coexist?

Ayurveda, despite being an age old system of medicine, has continued to face constant skepticism by the world. As scandals emerge, the authenticity and validity of Ayurveda is further questioned. Recently, the famous Baba Ramdev, who is well known for his Patanjali Ayurved products, was exposed for disseminating false information, claiming his products can cure serious ailments. He urged his audience to stop consuming synthetic medications, calling it poisonous and to begin utilizing these products, stating that they could cure illnesses such as cancer. Issues like this puts Ayurveda in a negative spotlight as well known, influential figures destroy the credibility of age old systems. This is also especially harmful because the world is not familiar with concepts preached by Ayurveda, therefore serious misconceptions arise, leading to mass skepticism.

Aside from events that help in destroying the reputation, there are certain concerns that arise when the topic of Ayurveda is brought up. One major problem is the issue with standardization. Unlike modern western medicine, where treatments are standardized and dosages are precisely measured, Ayurvedic treatments vary significantly, as they have complicated mixtures of herbs, minerals and other natural substances and this lack of uniformity leads to different effectiveness and quality in the results. While the issues with standardization addressed contribute to the validity of Ayurveda, I also believe that Ayurveda approaches treatment on a more personal level, designed for each person's Prakriti, which can limit the extent of standardization within this system.

Another significant problem is the lack of rigorous scientific research and clinical trials conducted, that supports Ayurvedic treatments. Additionally, Ayurvedic products are not regulated as strictly as conventional pharmaceuticals which again contributes to its view as an unreliable system. Cultural bias is also prevalent. As human beings, we are prone to have biased views , and western medical communities may be more skeptical of treatments that originate outside of the western scientific tradition. According to me however, what is truly harmful are the massive misconceptions surrounding Ayurveda. Some practitioners may make exaggerated claims about the benefits of Ayurveda, which can lead to unrealistic expectations and potential harm if people forego conventional treatments for serious conditions, as is the case with Baba Ramdev. Furthermore, people fail to understand that Ayurveda deals with holistic treatment. It's a lifestyle that recommends how one should live a healthy life, rather than just consuming certain medications and "curing" an illness.

In a conversation with an Ayurvedic doctor (Appendix A) who had studied this system of medicine intensively, I began to understand that while Ayurveda's role in modern society has evolved, the existence of Ayurveda, within the landscape of western medicine, would still remain to be an unlikely occurrence. During our discussion, she mentioned how the field of Ayurveda is evolving and gaining recognition beyond its origins in India. Although it is initially practiced primarily in India, Ayurveda has now found acceptance in various countries across the globe. European countries such as Germany, as well as Canada, and some Asian nations including Nepal, and Bangladesh, have embraced Ayurveda. While it may not yet be recognized as an official system of medicine in these countries, it has gained traction in the private sector, with many Ayurvedic practitioners operating there. Research and organization within Ayurveda are also advancing. The WHO has acknowledged Ayurveda as a system of medicine and has worked to standardize terminologies to bridge language barriers, as many traditional texts are in Sanskrit. The WHO established the Global Centre for Traditional Medicine (GCFTM) in India to assist other countries in standardizing Ayurvedic treatments. In the UK, for example, there are now associations offering Ayurvedic courses, including a five-and-a-half-year program or a diploma in Ayurveda. These courses are recognized and accredited, reflecting a growing interest in and acceptance of Ayurvedic principles.

In the past, those who sought to pursue degrees in Ayurveda, in the past had to learn about physiology, that is a part of the Ayurvedic curriculum in hospitals that practiced western medicine because there were limited institutions for specialized Ayurvedic education. As a result, allopathic medicine remains dominant in many regions, overshadowing alternative practices. Additionally, Ayurvedic supplements, which include herbs like Brahmi for brain function and Ashwagandha for immune support, skin care, and hair health, are increasingly available in Western countries without the need for a prescription. Many people in these countries are choosing Ayurvedic supplements over modern vitamin tablets, contributing to their popularity and sales in the Western market.

However, despite the progress made, Ayurveda and Western medicine still clash. Ayurvedic procedures differ significantly from Western medical procedures and the primary difference lies in the medications employed. Ayurveda relies entirely on plant-based herbal remedies, while Western medicine often uses synthetic drugs and pharmaceuticals. Another key difference is in the approach to treatment. Western medicine typically focuses on treating symptoms, while Ayurveda aims to diagnose and address the root causes of health issues, rather than just alleviating symptoms. Thus, the coexistence of these medical systems is unlikely, even in India. Allopathic medicine dominates the medical world and is mostly given precedence over

Ayurveda and other alternative systems, including homeopathy. Allopathic medicine has established itself as the primary system due to its capacity for immediate effects through its treatment and medications. On the other hand, alternative medicines, such as Ayurveda, generally offer gradual, long-term solutions and are considered complementary rather than competing systems.

Despite the increasing acceptance of Ayurveda across the world, challenges still remain, such as issues regarding the standardization of treatments, scientific validation, and regulatory practices. Additionally scandals, such as those involving Baba Ramdev, can damage the credibility of Ayurveda, leading to widespread misconceptions and skepticism. The integration of Ayurveda into the global medical landscape, while advancing, remains constrained by the dominance of Western medicine. To put it in simple words, the coexistence of Ayurveda and Western medicine is quite difficult due to the inherent differences in their approach to treatment.

Appendix A

The doctor I interviewed is based in London, having completed her education and training in India. She practiced Ayurveda for several years before relocating to London and moving on to research.

INTERVIEW TRANSCRIPT

Question 1:

What inspired you to become an Ayurvedic doctor?

Answer:

Growing up, I have always wanted to become a doctor. My parents are doctors so I grew up in that environment. I have always dreamed of becoming a doctor and helping patients, curing diseases. After I reached high school, in grade 12, I found medicine to be very intense, and not the kind of treatment I aimed to follow. Ayurveda addresses every disease from its root which fascinated me. It didn't just address the diseases but also directed us on how to live and have a healthy lifestyle.

Question 2:

Can you tell me about the kind of educational background and training you received to be an Ayurvedic doctor?

Answer:

To become an Ayurvedic doctor, I pursued a 5.5 year long degree in India, which was essentially 4.5 years of academic study followed by a year internship. Prior to my batch, the course duration was 3 professional years, but ours changed to 4.5 years. The syllabus remained largely the same and this was how it was structured, more or less, in the 3 year degree: In the first year, we learned Sanskrit, as a good understanding of the language is essential for studying Ayurveda since all the seminal texts are written in Sanskrit. This year also covered basic medicine, including physiology and anatomy with Sanskrit terminology, along with the foundational principles of Ayurveda, as outlined in the Ashtanga Hridaya. The second year focused on the first part of the Charaka Samhita, emphasizing Ayurvedic pharmacology, where I studied medicinal plants, the preparation of medicines, pathology, diagnostics, toxicology, and forensic medicine. In the third year, I completed the second volume of the Charaka Samhita and specialized in various clinical fields such as, but not limited to surgery, pediatrics, ENT, dentistry, OBGYN, and general medicine, as well as preventive medicine. The internship involves rotations across different specialties, including a one-month rural posting and practical experience in labor and some surgeries at government hospitals.

Question 3:

What additional studies did you pursue to be a practicing Ayurvedic doctor
based in London?

Answer:

No additional training is required per se, however you would have to join UK
associations that support Ayurveda. You can either practice privately or join a
clinic which practices Ayurveda.

Question 4:

How has your practice of Ayurveda influenced your own health and
wellbeing?

Answer:

What you learn first is the basic principle, which is maintaining the health of
healthy people and healing the ones suffering from problemsIt taught me how
to live a healthy life. I learned how to maintain my health, tackling problems
that I encountered daily such as anxiety, stress and insomnia. The two main
things that Ayurveda especially helped me in was with sleep deprivation. For
several years I struggled, and because of this insomnia, I had a mental fog: I
struggled to focus and had difficulty in concentration, often forgetting things
and lacking mental clarity. Through ayurveda, I learned that medicine is not
just the answer for these problems, rather, I needed to bring about a lifestyle
change, in a way that would give me peaceful sleep. The two procedures

Vamana and Virechana, intense processes that improve immunity and sleep without requiring medications. I also began eating healthy and regularly exercising such as running, walking in the evening, yoga, and meditation which helped with my sleep as well. I also had PCOS when I was younger and after implementing Ayurveda treatment processes my PCOS improved, I reduced weight as a result and my irregular menstruations improved with 28 days interval between each.

Question 5:

Can you share a few stories where Ayurvedic treatment made a significant impact on patients' wellbeing?

Answer:

I had patients who were around 19 or 20 years of age and married, coming for problems related to infertility. Their main problems were not caused due to infertility but because they had PCOS. I advised on implementing lifestyle changes such as exercising for 150 minutes every week, focus on their diet, such as having a more nutritious meal with more fiber and protein, as well as Univasthi which is the treatment of the uterus (strengthens the muscles and layers). Most of them were relieved of infertility. I had some patients come for problems from chronic illnesses such as diabetes. Began with addressing the symptoms, and if the patient was healthy enough, I recommended Shodhana therapies, and if they weren't healthy enough, treatment began with lifestyle changes and internal therapies.

Question 6:

How do you diagnose a patient in Ayurveda?

Answer:

When a patient comes, I first learn about the patient– their environment, their lifestyle, their medical history (surgeries and medicines they take). I then understand the disease, and in order to do so, I ask them to explain their symptoms, what they feel, their pain and their pain level. Next, physical examinations take place and the diagnostic examinations. You need to first understand the patient and then understand the disease. In order to understand the patient, you need to identify their Prakriti and then identify the nature of the disease– whether its Vataja, Pittaja or Kaphaja. For example, if the wound is dry, it's Vata; if it's slimy, it's Kapha; and if it has pus, it's Pitta. The line of treatments is then chosen accordingly.

Question 7:

What is Ayurveda's approach to chronic illnesses?

Answer:

Whenever a disease occurs, our body's immune system fights back. But when there is a chronic disease, our body is not able to bring back that normality. We consider the digestive fire, and chronic imbalance of doshas. Ayurveda seeks to bring back the digestive fire (boost immune system) and second is to bring back dosha balance. This is the general understanding of health. This is not just a symptomatic treatment, but also to understand the root cause of the disease, understand the Prakriti and assess it and then identify the Prakriti of the disease. Then we administer Shodhana therapies (Panchamukha therapies) and Shamana. We address Ahara and Vihara, and prescribe herbs and medications. For example, in Diabetes which is Kaphaja/Vataja disease, we address by administering Shodhana first (either Vamana or Basti) and then after purification, palliative care (changes in diet- for this particular disease we would ask the patient to avoid all types of fat and carbohydrates and include more protein and fiber). Lifestyle changes are to stay more active: engage in physical exercise in order to avoid a sedentary lifestyle

Question 8:

What are some common therapies used in Ayurveda? What are herbs and minerals

Answer:

There are three types of medicinal preparations: herbal medicines, medicines prepared from toxic plants and mineral preparations, also known as rasa preparations. Triphala, Brahmi, Tulsi and Amla are some herbs used as medicines. Toxic plants are purified before they are used as medicines, which includes Vatsanabha for arthritis, and Thanga (cannabis indica) to relieve pain and psychological disorders. For rasa preparation, there is the bhasma preparation, or the ashes preparation to make minerals/metals safe to consume as medicines, which includes Swarna (gold) , Rajat (silver), Tamra (copper), and Kajhulcc (mercury and sulfur).

Common therapies are Shodhana (purification), which includes all the therapies in panchaka; and Shamana (palliative therapies) which has all the internal (medicinal herbs consumed orally) and external applications (lepa or a herbal paste applied to skin).

Question 9:

How do you see the field of Ayurveda evolving?

Answer:

India was the only country accepting it, however, now, there are other countries such as Germany, Switzerland, Canada, and some Asian places, including Nepal, Bangladesh, Indonesia and Russia. It is not the main system of medicine, but it is accepted in the private sector. The WHO has recognized it as a system of medicine, and standardized terminologies to help countries understand principles (there is a language barrier as textbooks are in sanskrit). The WHO has also established a center in India, the GCFTM which helps other countries standardize treatments. Now, there are associations that can be found in the UK where they teach Ayurvedic courses (5.5 years or a diploma in

Ayurveda– accredited courses in other countries). People also consume supplementary medicines such as Brahmi tablets for your brain, and Ashwagandha for immunity. Many people consume Ayurvedic supplements instead of modern vitamin tablets, and these are big sellers in western countries.

Question 10:

Do you work with Western practitioners, and when do you recommend patients to Western practitioners?

Answer:

Yes. One time, a patient came to me with severe pain in his arm as he fell down and fractured it. If the fracture was just a hairline one, I would have been able to implement fracture treatment. If it is more than that however, allopathic modern hospitals are required. Another patient came with a severe dislocation. The patient was muscular, so it was difficult to set the bone. The patient was suffering from severe pain, so I referred them to allopathic practitioners.

Question 11:

How is Ayurvedic procedure different from Western medical procedure?

Answer:

The main difference is in the medicines. Modern medicines use chemicals whereas Ayurveda uses natural resources, such as, with herbal medicines. In modern medicine, they begin by treating symptoms, however in Ayurveda they diagnose and address the root cause of the disease.

Question 12:

How is Ayurveda integrated with modern medicine within the landscape of modern healthcare?

Answer:

Ayurveda was not accepted as a system of medicine before, however now, it's gaining popularity. It is now a second choice of treatment with scientific research going on, with research collaborations and therapy co-collaborations. Ayurvedic medicine is being accepted for pain management, as well as for recovery and rehabilitation, and even in postnatal care. There are ongoing standardisations, such as standardized formulations for Brahmi tablets, Ashwagandha tablets, and more. Ayurveda may not be the first choice of treatment, but it is the best after the first. Integrating Ayurvedic principles can help in maintaining health and preventing diseases before they require more intensive medical intervention.

The question on whether Ayurveda and Western medicine can exist together is a political question. I believe it would be a difficult reality as there is always one system that wants to dominate the other, with allopathy always having an upper hand. Systems such as Ayurveda, and homeopathy are all considered alternatives. Allopathic medicine will dominate as it has surgeries and medicines with immediate effects whereas alternatives have medicines that are effective gradually, over a long term period.

Question 13:

What are some common misconceptions about Ayurveda that you encounter at work and outside?

Answer:

The first misconception is that it is only purely based on herbal medicines. That is not true as it includes toxic plants, and minerals as well. The second is that it does not have any side effects. Some mineral preparations should be administered with proper care and supervision, unlike herbal medicines. Ayurveda is not instantaneous. It requires time and needs patience for the medicine to act in our body. People assume that it is not based on research or science, however, there is research going on in Indian and foreign universities, based on treatments and herbal medicines and certain drugs. Finally, it is important to note that Ayurveda is a lifestyle not a treatment. The approach to ayurveda is very different as it doesn't just address the symptoms but the root cause. Some people think that medicines are the only things needed. It is about the lifestyle changes, and along with that the medicines.

Appendix B: References

Ayurveda. (n.d.). *Types of Diagnosis*. [online] Available at:
https://www.keralatourism.org/ayurveda/diagnosis/five-
types#:~:text=The%20five%20main%20types%20of.

Ayurveda. (2021). *What is Ayurveda? Introduction & Guide | The Ayurvedic
Institute*. [online] Available at: https://ayurveda.com/ayurveda-a-brief-
introduction-and-guide/.

Bhavana, K. and Shreevathsa (2014). Medical geography in Charaka Samhita.
AYU (An International Quarterly Journal of Research in Ayurveda), 35(4),
p.371. doi:https://doi.org/10.4103/0974-8520.158984.

Birla Ayurveda (2023). *Ways Of Diagnosis In Ayurveda | Birla Ayurveda*.
[online] Birla Healthcare Ayurveda Pvt. Ltd. Available at:
https://birlaayurveda.co.in/ways-of-diagnosis-in-ayurveda/.

Cronkleton, E. (2022). *Vata dosha: Diet, meaning, characteristics, and more.*
[online] www.medicalnewstoday.com. Available at:
https://www.medicalnewstoday.com/articles/vata-dosha#what-is-it.

Dabur. (n.d.). *Amla Benefits*. [online] Available at:
https://www.dabur.com/ayurveda/ayurvedic-medicinal-plants/amla.

Dabur. (2015a). *Tulsi*. [online] Available at:

https://www.dabur.com/ayurveda/ayurvedic-medicinal-plants/tulsi-benefits-

and-medicinal-uses#:~:text=Tulsi%20is%20an%20age%2Dold.

Dabur. (2015b). *What is Vata Dosha?* [online] Available at:

https://www.dabur.com/blog/doshas/what-vata-dosha.

Davidson, K. (2020). *What Are the Ayurveda Doshas? Vata, Kapha, and Pitta

Explained*. [online] Healthline. Available at:

https://www.healthline.com/nutrition/vata-dosha-pitta-dosha-kapha-

dosha#ayurveda-doshas.

Dr Manasa (2016a). *Acharya Charaka - Work, Samhita, Legacy, Chapters,

Description*. [online] Easy Ayurveda. Available at:

https://www.easyayurveda.com/2016/07/21/acharya-charaka-work-samhita-

legacy/#charaka_samhita.

Dr Manasa (2016b). *Acharya Vagbhata: Work, Text Books, Legacy, Amazing

Facts*. [online] Easy Ayurveda. Available at:

https://www.easyayurveda.com/2016/08/21/acharya-vagbhata/.

Dr Manasa (2016c). *Lord Dhanwantari 'The God of Ayurveda'*. [online] Easy

Ayurveda. Available at: https://www.easyayurveda.com/2016/09/12/lord-

dhanwantari-the-god-of-ayurveda/#dhanwantari

Dr Raghuram and Dr Manasa (2017). *Nidana: Meaning, Word Derivation, Definition*. [online] Easy Ayurveda. Available at: https://www.easyayurveda.com/2017/06/18/nidana-meaning-word-derivation-definition/.

Dr Raghuram and Dr Manasa (2018). *Purvaroopa Definition, Types, Benefits Of Its Knowledge, Features*. [online] Easy Ayurveda. Available at: https://www.easyayurveda.com/2018/04/16/purvaroopa-pragroopa/.

Dr Raghuram and Dr Manasa (2019). *Upashaya Anupashaya - Pacifying And Non-Pacifying Factors Of Disease*. [online] Easy Ayurveda. Available at: https://www.easyayurveda.com/2019/10/25/upashaya-anupashaya/.

e-Samhita - National Institute of Indian Medical Heritage. (n.d.). *Susrutasamhita*. [online] Available at: https://niimh.nic.in/ebooks/esushruta/?mod=home&con=pro.

e-Vagbhata - Institute of Ayurveda and Integrative Medicine (I-AIM). (2024). *About Samhita*. [online] Available at: https://vedotpatti.in/samhita/Vag/vagbhata/?mod=home&con=as.

Encyclopedia Britannica. (n.d.). *Sushruta | Indian surgeon*. [online] Available at: https://www.britannica.com/biography/Sushruta.

Guha, A. (2016). *Where does Ayurveda come from? | taking charge of your health & wellbeing*. [online] Taking Charge of Your Health & Wellbeing.

Available at: https://www.takingcharge.csh.umn.edu/where-ayurveda-come-from.

Hasan, M.R., Alotaibi, B.S., Althafar, Z.M., Mujamammi, A.H. and Jameela, J. (2023). An Update on the Therapeutic Anticancer Potential of Ocimum sanctum L.: 'Elixir of Life'. *Molecules*, [online] 28(3), p.1193. doi:https://doi.org/10.3390/molecules28031193.

Johns Hopkins Medicine. (2024). *Ayurveda.* [online] Available at: https://www.hopkinsmedicine.org/health/wellness-and-prevention/ayurveda#:~:text=Ayurveda%2C%20a.

Loukas, M., Lanteri, A., Ferrauiola, J., Tubbs, R.S., Maharaja, G., Shoja, M.M., Yadav, A. and Rao, V.C. (2010). Anatomy in ancient India: a focus on the Susruta Samhita. *Journal of Anatomy*, 217(6), pp.646–650. doi:https://doi.org/10.1111/j.1469-7580.2010.01294.x.

Mapi. (2021). *Understanding the 5 Subdoshas of Kapha.* [online] Available at: https://mapi.com/blogs/articles/understanding-the-5-subdoshas-of-kapha.

Metz, H.-J. (2019). *Maharishi Ayurveda Gesundheits- und Seminarzentrum Bad Ems GmbH.* [online] Maharishi Ayurveda Health Centre Bad Ems. Available at: https://ayurveda-badems.com/the-five-subdoshas-of-pitta/.

Mollan, C. (2024). Baba Ramdev: The yoga guru under fire over Patanjali's 'natural cures'. *www.bbc.com.* [online] 18 Apr. Available at: https://www.bbc.com/news/world-asia-india-68816285.

Murthy, A.R. (1997). Dhanwantari: the God of Hindu medicine. *Bulletin of the Indian Institute of History of Medicine (Hyderabad),* [online] 27(1), pp.1–14. Available at: https://pubmed.ncbi.nlm.nih.gov/12572586/#:~:text=Abstract.

Nakshatra Ayurvedam. (2017). *Samhita.* [online] Available at: https://www.nakshatraayurvedam.com/samhita.html#:~:text=Laghu%20Trayi.

National Cancer Institute (2019). *NCI Dictionary of Cancer Terms.* [online] National Cancer Institute. Available at: https://www.cancer.gov/publications/dictionaries/cancer-terms/def/cerebrospinal-fluid.

Prasad, S. and Aggarwal, B.B. (2011). *Turmeric, the Golden Spice: From Traditional Medicine to Modern Medicine.* 2nd ed. [online] PubMed. Available at: https://www.ncbi.nlm.nih.gov/books/NBK92752/#:~:text=In%20Ayurvedic%20Opractices%2C%20turmeric%20is.

Sabatino, M., Murarka, P.V. and Shakti, P. (2022). *Aṣṭāṅga Hṛdayam and Aṣṭāṅga Saṃgraha: Compare and Contrast.* [online] History of Ayurveda. Available at: https://www.historyofayurveda.org/library/aga-hdayam-and-aga-sagraha-compare-and-contrast.

Shilpa, S. and Venkatesha Murthy, C.G. (2011). Understanding personality from Ayurvedic perspective for psychological assessment: A case. *Ayu,* [online] 32(1), pp.12–19. doi:https://doi.org/10.4103/0974-8520.85716.

Singh, N., Bhalla, M., De Jager, P. and Gilca, M. (2011). An Overview on Ashwagandha: A Rasayana (Rejuvenator) of Ayurveda. *African Journal of Traditional, Complementary and Alternative Medicines*, [online] 8(5S). doi:https://doi.org/10.4314/ajtcam.v8i5s.9.

Singh, V. (2017). Sushruta: The father of surgery. *National Journal of Maxillofacial Surgery*, [online] 8(1), p.1. doi:https://doi.org/10.4103/njms.njms_33_17.

Somatheeram Ayurvedic Health Resort. (n.d.). *The Pitta type in Ayurveda.* [online] Available at: https://somatheeram.org/en/pitta/.

Sri Sri College of Ayurvedic Science & Research Hospital. (2023). *6 Stages Of Disease- Navigating to the Path of Wellness.* [online] Available at: https://srisriayurvedahospital.org/6-stages-of-disease/#:~:text=%E2%80%9CSamprapti%E2%80%9D%20refers%20to%20the%20concept.

Templeton, K. (n.d.). *About Pitta.* [online] yogainternational.com. Available at: https://yogainternational.com/article/view/about-pitta/.

Thakar, V. (2010). Historical development of basic concepts of Ayurveda from Veda up to Samhita. *AYU (An International Quarterly Journal of Research in Ayurveda)*, 31(4), p.400. doi:https://doi.org/10.4103/0974-8520.82024.

The Ayurvedic Clinic. (2019). *The Srotas Channnels of Circulation*. [online] Available at: https://www.theayurvedicclinic.com/the-srotas-or-channels-of-circulation/#:~:text=The%20doshas%20of%20the%20body,Maha%20%E2%80%93%20large%20or%20great).

The Editors of Encyclopedia Britannica (2014). Charaka-samhita | Indian medical text. In: *Encyclopædia Britannica*. [online] Available at: https://www.britannica.com/topic/Charaka-samhita.

Unnikrishnan, P.M., Shankar, D. and Unnikrishnan, P.M. (2004). 'The Materia Medica of Ayurveda', in Challenging the Indian Medical Heritage. Foundation Books (Environment and Development Series), pp. 40–62..

Upper Valley Yoga. (2016). *Udana Vayu: The Up Breath—Voice and Intention*. [online] Available at: https://www.uppervalleyyoga.com/blog/post-56.

Vikaspedia. (2024). *The Concept of Ahara (Diet) in Ayurveda*. [online] Available at: https://vikaspedia.in/health/ayush/ayurveda-1/ayurveda-based-dietary-guidelines-for-mental-disorders/the-concept-of-ahara-diet-in-ayurveda#:~:text=The%20preventive%20and%20curative%20aspects,Ashtavidha%20Ahara%20Vidhi%20Visesha%20Ayatana).

Wasatch Ayurveda & Yoga. (2019). *The Srotas: Channels of the Body - Wasatch Ayurveda & Yoga.* [online] Available at: https://www.wasatchayurvedaandyoga.com/srotas-channels-body/.

58

Acknowledgements

I would like to thank all those who supported me in completing this book. I extend my gratitude to my mentors and educators who helped guide my writing. I also appreciate the feedback I received from my early readers, which helped shape the final manuscript. A special thank you goes to the interview participant, who provided invaluable insights, clarified my doubts, and further enhanced my knowledge. I would also like to thank my family and friends for their encouragement throughout this journey. This project has not only deepened my understanding of Ayurveda but has also made me more eager to share what I've learned.

www.ingramcontent.com/pod-product-compliance
Lightning Source LLC
Chambersburg PA
CBHW040134150726
48005CB00015B/2502